DIY
Health Guide

DIY
Health Guide

Maria Jevtic BSc (Hons)

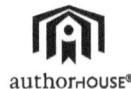

authorHOUSE®

AuthorHouse™
1663 Liberty Drive
Bloomington, IN 47403
www.authorhouse.com
Phone: 1-800-839-8640

First published by AuthorHouse   08/11/2011

ISBN: 978-1-4567-8519-2 (sc)
ISBN: 978-1-4567-8520-8 (ebk)

Printed in the United States of America

Any people depicted in stock imagery provided by Thinkstock are models, and such images are being used for illustrative purposes only.
Certain stock imagery © Thinkstock.

This book is printed on acid-free paper.

Contents

None of the information in this book is intended as a substitute for medical advice. Always consult a registered medical doctor.

Introduction

With this guide I want to encourage you to take a large part of your health care into your own hands. I do not intend to make your life a misery, quite the opposite. I will show you how much of your health and happiness is of your own making.

There are many factors influencing your state of health, and in this guide I list the most important ones. Some factors are out of your hands, and I will let you know how to handle these. It is my belief that if you implement the measures discussed below, your health should improve. For this it does not matter what state of health you are in at present—whether you are in almost perfect health, you have some minor ailments, or you are seriously ill.

If there is only one idea to remember from this guide, it must be this:

> The more lifestyle measures you implement, the less you will need to use some form of medicine to help you with your symptoms.

Your Health Bank Account

I would like to start with this simple concept:

> Your body works like a bank account. Just as with money, you can pay in and you can take out. The way to stay in credit is to pay in more than you take out.

We are born with a certain fixed level of health; this is our credit. Many people call this our "constitution". This was given to us at conception. From then on we try to keep the account in credit. This is not easy when our constitutional health is continuously eroded by the onslaughts of pollution, infection, and emotional stress.

The good news is that we can protect ourselves. We can even improve on our constitutional health by using lifestyle and medical measures prudently and judiciously. In other words, it is within our power to build on our constitution and keep our health bank account strong and thriving. Please be aware that *some of the factors involved are not under our control*. In effect, however, this just means that we need to make an extra effort with the ones we do have control over.

The concept of a health bank account can simplify our daily lives enormously. Without becoming obsessed, we can keep an eye on our habits and attitudes and make sure that we engage more in positive ones than negative ones. This way, we should at least maintain our constitutional health.

Why can one person smoke and drink and still remain healthy, whereas another dies of lung cancer twenty years after having had just a couple of cigarettes? The explanation is to be found in their health bank accounts. *Overall*, the first person must have paid in more than he took out and so remained healthy. The second person did not continue to smoke, but the rest of his lifestyle was probably majorly health-eroding.

What exactly are those things that we call "health-eroding"? There is so much debate and controversy. Whom can we believe? Advice changes every few years too. My answer is: use your common sense. Read on and see for yourself whether you think I make sense to you. I am going to discuss the main areas that influence our health, and I will let you know the conclusions I have come to.

When I speak about health, I mean our emotional, mental, and physical health. I will also touch on spiritual health and give you my opinion on this controversial subject.

I will simplify my approach by stating that there are a number of basic building blocks that open the possibility of a disease-free life. Whether your life will in fact be disease-free or not depends on your original bank account balance and how much you pay in and take out. Please be aware that *some of the building blocks are not under your control*. To prevent your account from slipping towards chronic disease, you must therefore ensure that you do as much as you can in those areas that *are* under your control. For example: To protect against air pollution, you could make sure your diet contains an extraordinary amount of antioxidants to ward off the damage air pollution causes. Alternatively, you could use certain disciplines of alternative medicine (I will discuss these later) that have the power to stimulate your defences to provide protection.

Building Block 1: Nutrition

Nutrition is probably one of the most controversial and confusing topics. I therefore ask you to do nothing but use your common sense. Please keep an open mind and follow through my explanations.

Human beings are different from other animals. They can override their natural instinctive appetite and arrive at all sorts of strange convolutions when it comes to food.

Some people are guided by their cravings; they claim that if they crave something, that means their body must need it. Some are guided by their sense of ethics; they claim that certain foods are unhealthy, when in fact they feel morally guilty when eating them. Some people are routine driven and/ or addicted and cannot possibly imagine changing their food choices. Some people are supporters of the whole-food movement and eat what looks like bird food to others.

Where are you in this?

> You are of the species *Homo sapiens*. This species firmly established itself about 200,000 years ago and physically has not changed one bit since then. Our digestive system has not changed; our liver processes have not changed; our ability to use food and eliminate waste has not changed. Our body had perfectly evolved to eat a certain diet. It did so in the same way as everything else about us evolved to ensure the survival of the species. It did so in the same way as every other life form on this planet evolved. (Some life forms do disappear, but this is normally due to a sudden change in the environment which the life form cannot adapt to quickly enough.)

Back to Man.

Early *Homo sapiens* ate meat, fish, eggs, fruit, nuts, seeds, and any vegetable matter that seemed palatable and was non-toxic. There is no creature in nature that is not perfectly adapted to eating the diet they chose to eat. *Homo sapiens* was eating the perfect diet for the survival of the species.

The question is whether or not some other items can be added to this diet without paying a price!

Let me continue. We carried on eating this diet for 190,000 years until about 10,000 years ago.

Then something changed. We settled down and became farmers. We started drinking milk and eating cereals and pulses. Nothing else changed until about AD 1840, when we gradually began adding all sorts of non-food substances to our diet. Today in AD 2010, a lot of what we eat no Stone Age man would even recognise as food.

This change in our diet has taken place over 500 generations.

Have we changed our DNA or metabolism in 10,000 years? Definitely not.

But we have changed our diet.

The question is: Is this relevant to our quest for health?

To me it is, and all I'm reasonably asking of you is that you at least take this into consideration. Our present health crisis must have its roots somewhere, and diet may well be one of the major contributing factors.

Some people claim that a large proportion of our chronic disease states are related to having eaten a faulty diet over generations—a diet that we are not meant to eat and that has only been around for these last 500 generations.

Opponents say that the only reason we did not have chronic disease before 8000 BC is because we were killed off by accidents and wild animals well before we could have developed such diseases. And true enough, nowadays most adults begin noticing stubborn symptoms around the age of forty, well after many Stone Age people would have died.

We can discuss this forever, but unfortunately in the end we will believe what suits us individually (and we will find reasons for doing so).

To achieve a degree of clarity in our own minds, let's look at the question of diet from another angle. In the present dietary maze, are there any fundamental dietary principles from which we must not digress (too far and too often) in order to remain free of chronic disease?

My answer to this is yes.

I believe that regardless of where we came from and what Stone Age man used to eat, we now have enough knowledge to understand two scientifically established fundamental dietary principles. Sticking to these throughout our lives will—in my opinion—hold between fifty and seventy per cent of chronic disease at bay. This is not just because your body will get everything it needs and avoid a lot of food toxins. Eating this way will also protect you to a great extent from environmental pollution and other factors that are out of your control, such as radiation and damaging emotional stress.

Here are the two fundamental principles a healthy, disease-preventing diet must fulfil:

- **The diet must supply all the essential nutrients in required amounts.** (otherwise deficiency symptoms will set a slowly progressing disease state into motion).

- **The diet must provide more alkaline compounds to your body than acidic compounds** (otherwise a poorly alkalised system will set a slowly progressing disease state into motion).

Forget about the small issues such as meat, carbs, supplements, coffee, cholesterol, etc.

These issues are secondary to the two fundamental principles stated above. As long as your diet supplies your body with all you need *and* it is alkalizing your tissues, you can drink coffee, eat meat, have cholesterol, and you do not need supplements (except omega 3)!

Actually, you will find that when you apply these two principles, you will not have much room, tolerance, or need for coffee, alcohol, supplements (except omega 3), or any of the other controversial food items that nutritionists have been fighting over for decades. Your tummy will be full and satisfied, and your mind will turn to more interesting things than eating and drinking. You will have all the energy for your day-to-day activities and your regular exercise.

So let us explain in more detail what these two principles mean and what your ideal diet would look like.

Please follow my explanations below.

We need to eat a full set of nutrients in the required amounts.

The list of essential nutrients is undisputed, but required amounts are subject to controversy.

- **Protein:** Essential for making body structures and components as well as hormones and chemical messengers. Protein is needed to make body parts! Major sources of concentrated protein: meat, fish, eggs, pulses including soy, dairy, nuts.

- **Carbohydrate:** Our major source of energy. It is broken down into glucose and burned to enable chemical reactions and movement as well as mental processes. Major sources of concentrated carbohydrates: cereals, pulses, vegetables, fruit.

- **Fat:** Needed to insulate the body from cold, to insulate organs from mechanical damage, to make hormones, to provide fuel to some special parts such as the heart, to build the brain and nervous system, to build cell membranes. Major sources of fat: meat, fish, eggs, dairy, nuts, seeds, olives.

- **Fibre:** Needed to enable elimination of stool. Major sources of fibre: cereals, vegetables, fruit.

- **Vitamins:** Enable chemical reactions to take place. Needed by the immune system, for bones and teeth, for defence against pollution and sunlight, for energy release from glucose, and for just about every chemical reaction in the body. Major sources of vitamins: vegetables, fruit.

- **Minerals:** Enable chemical reactions to take place. Structural components in teeth, bones and other connective tissues. Needed for blood sugar balance, immune system, oxygen delivery, and harvesting of energy from food, to name a few.

- **Water:** Provides a medium for chemical reactions. Enables waste elimination through urine, stool, and sweat.

- **Antioxidants/phytochemicals**: Defend against pollution, help detoxification of body's own waste. Major sources: fruit, vegetables, some seeds and mushrooms.

Nutrient deficiencies lead to progressive disease states. This means illness will creep up on you slowly but surely, because all nutrients are essential for keeping your body in good working order!

Certain foods are vitamin—and mineral—poor or produce a net loss of these nutrients during their processing in the body. So whilst you are gaining minerals from cereals, the processing of cereals uses up more than you gained. Therefore you end up with a deficiency of minerals if you eat too many cereals and too few vegetables (which are high in minerals and vitamins). People who eat diets high in cereals are usually deficient in magnesium, zinc, manganese, and iron, as well as the vitamin B complex.

Apart from nutrient content, we also need to choose foods according to their acid or alkaline producing properties. This is because we require alkaline tissues in order to remain healthy and free of progressive disease states.

Most foods are acid-producing. Only vegetables and fruit leave alkalinity in your tissues. In order to receive enough alkalinity, more alkaline foods (in dry weight) must be eaten than acid-producing ones.

Acid-providing foods are highly concentrated, whereas vegetables and fruit contain a lot of water to carry their alkalinity in. This means that weight for weight you have to eat a lot more vegetables and fruit in order to balance out the acidity gained from acid-producing foods.

It so happens that foods delivering alkalinity to our tissues also deliver a rich variety of phytochemicals, plus all the vitamin and mineral we need in plentiful supply. These foods are vegetables and fruit.

Regardless of what else you eat, three quarters of your daily foods must come from fresh vegetables and fruit, or you will enter a progressive disease state because of accumulating acidity and mineral/vitamin/phytochemical deficiency.

The longer you cook fresh vegetables, the more nutrients you will lose and the less alkalinity they will provide. Steaming and stir-frying are therefore the best cooking methods.

Vegetables and fruit eaten in these large amounts will supply all the carbohydrates you need for energy/glucose. You will also get all the fibre you need. This makes it entirely unnecessary to eat cereals as a source of carbohydrates and fibre.

You now only need to add a source of healthy fats and proteins to your daily diet.

Healthy fats must include essential omega 3 and 6 fatty acids, which are in poor supply even if you eat your three servings of fish per week!

6

Everyone needs to supplement these to prevent problems with the immune system, nervous system, hormones, and skin.

Protein can be sourced from animals or plants, but plant protein comes (in my opinion) with more problems than animal protein. One problem is that plant protein (which comes mostly from pulses) predisposes us to anaemia, digestive system problems, and net mineral loss. Dairy protein comes with undesirable carcinogenic growth hormone factors. This subject is controversial, and so I will not go into it much further. Besides, the question of meat and dairy consumption is secondary to need to fulfil the two dietary truths stated above.

However:

- Meat does not have to be unhealthy as long as it is lean, unprocessed, organic, and not char-grilled.

- On the other hand, animal husbandry comes with heavy moral/ ethical burdens; for this reason many people perhaps rightly consider meat ***not*** to be an ideal food.

To summarize: your ideal diet should definitely consist of three quarters vegetables and fruit in order to guarantee alkalinity and mineral/vitamin/ phytochemical and fibre supply. You then need to add one quarter protein and healthy fat (including omega 3 and 6 oils). Carbohydrates and fibre are supplied in sufficient quantities by vegetables and fruit.

Vegetables and fruit are only healthy if they are fresh. No canned, frozen, or processed varieties please. Stay away from denatured and processed foods in general.

Human beings are very resilient. You must break your ideal diet sometimes just to make sure you are not becoming obsessed, fussy, or rigid in your attitude. The occasional transgression into a paradise of dairy, deserts, or carbs will do you no harm.

Water is the most ideal drink. Ordinary tea and coffee should be restricted to one cup per day, as these stimulants strain your blood sugar balance and make you lose minerals. They also add to your toxic burden.

Herbal teas, green tea, and high quality fruit juices are tolerable as long as you don't overindulge in them. Alcoholic beverages (except beer) are actually for the most part alkaline-producing and therefore not too bad—in moderation! I set the limit at four units per week. Fizzy drinks and energy drinks, as well as poor-quality fruit juices, are definitely health-eroding.

Children should never be allowed to drink ordinary tea, coffee, alcohol, or fizzy drinks. Once your child is hooked on any of these, you will have trouble getting them off, so it is best never to start. Cola drinks contain far too much sugar, carcinogenic chemicals, addictive substances, blood sugar disrupters, stimulants, colourings, flavourings, etc. Fanta and other lemonades are not much better.

If you want to use food or drink as a treat for your child, let them have a hot chocolate or some other honest sweet item, such as a good quality ice cream, continental chocolate, or homemade cake. At least you know what is in those, and you will pretty much limit the damage to plain sugar and fat.

Beware of artificial sweeteners and glutamates, MSG, and other flavour enhancers. These are extremely unhealthy for your nervous system. They are contained in vegetarian meat-substitute products, Asian foods, Oriental foods, many processed and packaged foods, drinks, cakes, diet goods, and so on. Stay away as much as possible!

Summary

Three quarters of your diet must be vegetables and fruit. The rest will self-regulate to a great extent. I suggest adding just meat or fish and eggs, plus olive oil and fish oil (omega 3 and 6).

There is no doubt about the two dietary principles. They cannot be disregarded without paying a price in terms of your overall health. A car cannot run without fuel; you cannot run without alkalising, nutrient-rich food.

Acidic foods	Neutral foods	Alkaline foods
meat, fish		
eggs, pulses	milk	vegetables
soy(!)	yoghurt	fruit
cereals	fats	wine
cheese		

Supplements

Vitamin and mineral supplements can be useful in two ways:

- to make good any nutrient deficiencies in our diet

- as therapeutic agents to increase specific chemical reactions in our body which are necessary for healing

In an ideal world, we would get all the vitamins, minerals, essential fats, and phytochemicals we need from our diet. If you follow the diet laid out above, you will not be short in any nutrients except perhaps calcium (for a growing child) and essential fats (omega 3). I therefore recommend everyone to supplement their diet with a high quality fish oil supplement. I also recommend a high quality calcium supplement for children who do not eat dairy.

People who live in a much polluted inner-city environment should also take a high strength anti-oxidant supplement. (See Building Block 6 below.)

People who do not eat a nutrient-rich diet as described above may need to supplement specific vitamins and minerals. A must are all the B vitamins, magnesium, and zinc.

Any other supplements are a waste of time and money, unless you are very unwell and/or need to make good a backlog of deficiencies. If you *are* chronically ill or have recurring problems, I recommend you consult a nutritional therapist (See Building Block 7 below.)

Nutritional therapy uses specific nutrients such as magnesium, zinc, and vitamin B, as well as glandular and herbal extracts to bring about healing in your body. In this case, the prescribed supplements are therapeutic agents and should only be taken for a limited time as specified by a practitioner.

If you find yourself slipping down the slippery road of taking more and more supplements on a daily basis, stop and take stock! You are probably emotionally or mentally addicted.

There is a new condition called "orthorexia", which is the state of being obsessively concerned about your diet and making your own life (and probably that of your family) a misery because of this. There is a fine line between being a responsible eater and being obsessed, so please slow down and ask yourself occasionally where you are in this spectrum.

Going back to our concept of a health bank account, it is important to remember that if your diet is not ideal, you can make up this short-coming and keep your bank account thriving *to some extent* by paying more attention to the other building blocks. For example, if you decide you wanted to drink more alcohol on a regular basis than the recommended four units per week, you could instead sleep more hours than is commonly necessary, or you could see a homeopath and let him or her prescribe a liver-supporting tincture to prevent your liver from becoming progressively over worked.

Let's therefore have a look at the next building block of health.

Building Block 2:
Sleep and Rest

Humans need to sleep and rest. There is nothing heroic or admirable about needing little sleep or never taking a holiday or even a tea break. Don't fall into the trap of believing reports you hear about some amazingly rare people who sleep less than three hours per night and carry on regardless. This is an exception and may not even be a true representation of the whole picture. Do you know how many cups of coffee per day these people drink? Are they having energy drinks? Do you know how many sugary stimulants they eat? Do you know whether they are perfectly healthy or whether they perhaps have continuous headaches, sinus problems, digestive upsets, and the like? Do you follow through and check how healthy they are ten years down the line?

Please do not fall for these stories without keeping in mind that there is a whole part of the story you do not know.

At this point I would make one concession. Doing what you enjoy and what fulfils you completely will give you seemingly endless energy without negative short-term or long-term effects.

This is why some people can carry on with very little sleep or rest. But this is an exception, because most of us are bound by our daily chores and financial duties.

Why do we need to sleep?

Nobody knows for sure, but here are some facts that help us understand the importance of getting enough sleep.

- When we sleep our conscious mind is switched off. This saves an enormous amount of energy.

- Switching off the conscious mind also allows our nervous system to go into its "maintenance mode". This mode enables the body to restore balance to all its background functions, such as digestion, blood sugar control, waste elimination, and so on.

- These background functions go on all the time, but during sleep the body gets a slot of several hours to perform "housekeeping" as its main activity.

- Physical growth takes place during sleep, which is why children need more sleep than adults.

- Our biorhythms are aligned with the hormone cortisol secreted by the adrenal glands. Cortisol secretion begins to rise at 4 a.m., and this gradually wakes us. Cortisol secretion begins to fall at 4 p.m., and this gradually makes us sleepy.

- People who go to sleep after midnight on a regular basis either cause or react to a shift in their cortisol levels. In either case, their cortisol secretion remains high after 4 p.m. and remains low after 4 a.m. This shift causes poor ability to wake in the morning and high energy in the evening, preventing sleep.

- This would not be a problem if we did not have to get up early—or earlier than our cortisol levels want us to. If we feel tired and listless in the morning, we will use stimulants to get us going. These artificially raise our cortisol and do so continuously for several hours at a time. We end up with an even poorer ability to wind down at night, causing a loss of sleep. Thus we enter a vicious cycle that keeps us sleep-deprived and reliant on stimulants to perform.

I personally believe that a minimum seven hours of uninterrupted sleep are necessary to perform the most pressing maintenance work on a daily basis. Some adults need up to nine hours.

What about resting and taking time out?

> In my opinion, in many people the conscious mind can actively interfere with the body's rebalancing efforts! When we are awake, our mind does not stop. It chatters on and on, even while we are doing something else. But much of our level of health depends on *what* the mind is saying and how good we are at stopping it from interfering with our basic health.

How does the mind interfere?

> To simplify, if your mind is continuously playing the "hurry" song—"must get this done, must get that done, I'm late, too much to do", and so on—these thoughts will create a low-level physical stress response. When the body is in this stress response, it cannot perform background functions such as elimination, digestion, etc. very well. This will leave a backlog of work to do, which will never decrease unless you switch of that mind and . . . sleep! This process is very subtle, and most of us will never be aware of it at all.

> Another example of an interfering mind would be the mind that is playing the "must achieve" song—"have to finish, have to impress, not good enough, what if I fail, he is better than me, and so on". This mind also creates tension similar to the stress response of the previous case. During this tense state, the body will perform poorly on background maintenance work, therefore needing more sleep later.

By switching the conscious mind off or by letting it play positive messages that have a stress-reducing effect, the body can maintain and repair itself in peace.

Meditation and prayer (or simply lying under a palm tree and watching the waves) are techniques and situations during which we can observe our mind's chatter and become aware of its quality. Once we are aware, we can learn to let negative chatter go and even employ positive self-talk to improve our stress response. Learning this may take special instruction by a specialist in NLP (neurolinguistic programming) or any other therapy that addresses the mind.

What about the subconscious?

> We said that while you are resting and sleeping, your body can go into maintenance mode.
>
> Meanwhile, during the day and the night, your subconscious mind is playing its own song. It may be directly opposed to the more conscious one I have mentioned above, and this discrepancy may be a source of major health problems.
>
> There is no way of switching the subconscious off, but it is possible to access and re-programme it through various techniques such as NLP and hypnosis.
>
> There is another way to access some of our subconscious: it reveals itself in our dreams—not in **all** dreams, but definitely in **some**, especially through recurring themes. Recognising recurring themes and working out their meaning can be a valuable tool in improving our energy and therefore our health. There are several disciplines of health care that work with dreams and the subconscious mind, such as Jungian psychotherapy.

Please note that too much or too little dreaming is a symptom of imbalance. If you do not have any other symptoms, this is nothing to worry about. If you do have other symptoms, I would look into it. It may be a simple vitamin deficiency, or it may be caused by excessive alcohol consumption. In the case of no dreaming, you may be putting a subconscious emotional block in place to protect yourself from unpleasant messages coming to your conscious mind. In the case of excessive and disturbing dreaming, you may be compensating. In other words, you may be doing at night what you should be doing or want to be doing during the day.

Whichever it is, I believe that a moderate dream life can enrich our experience and may even help us to understand ourselves and the world around us at another level.

But even if you do not wish to go into the more wishy-washy areas, such as dreams or your subconscious, please take one piece of advice:

Sleep, sleep, sleep.

Sleeping is not a waste of time. It actually enhances your waking hours and adds years to your life. Sleep can cure influenza and infections. Sleep rebalances bad moods and emotional upheavals. Sleep rejuvenates.

Time in bed is time well spent. Seven to nine hours per night is all you need.

Night Shifts

Please avoid these at all costs, as night shifts upset your cortisol rhythm (see above) and so may increase the risk of blood sugar problems and metabolic diseases such as diabetes. If you cannot avoid working at night or only have to do night shifts periodically, please be extra careful in other ways, such as diet and exercise. I also strongly recommend seeing a homeopath and/or chiropractor regularly to keep your nervous system and hormonal balance working. For people who cross time-zones regularly, homeopathy and chiropractic may help you adjust quickly and without much trouble, taking the stress away.

A Special Note on Children

Children need to sleep. Regular hours and long periods of uninterrupted sleep are paramount for their general health, immune system, and development.

If you have a child under the age of ten who is a poor sleeper, i.e. goes to sleep late, wakes frequently, needs to go to the bathroom, etc., I recommend that you investigate the causes and take appropriate measures. It may be that there are actual reasons, or it may simply be habit.

Some babies never learn how to soothe themselves to sleep or how to go back to sleep after waking at night. I recommend a book by Richard Ferber called *Solve Your Child's Sleep Problems.* This book explains all matters around sleep and helps you to teach your baby or toddler to soothe him or herself to sleep.

Some parents have unrealistic expectations of their children's sleep routine. A 7 p.m. bedtime is far too early for most children aged six and above. If you insist on too early bedtimes and your child is not able to sleep at that time, you may set a pattern for habitual insomnia and sleep problems in later life. Equally, expecting your eleven year old to sleep at 8 p.m. is a disaster and will again lead to poor sleeping patterns and insomnia later on.

Too early bedtimes are also a problem when it comes to the ability to concentrate at school. If your child wakes at 5.30 a.m. because they went to bed too early, they will have been up and about for three hours before school even starts! Of course they will be tired and cranky when you pick them up at 3 p.m., and probably they cannot concentrate for most of their lessons after lunch.

I suggest that you read Richard Ferber's book to familiarise yourself with average sleep requirements and then try to retrain your child's sleep patterns as gently as possible. Children need to be fresh and rested for school, and they need to acquire a happy and healthy sleep pattern.

Building Block 3:
Exercise and Activity

Back to our Stone Age man. *Homo sapiens* evolved as a hunter-gatherer. Much of his day was spent in activity. He engaged in many hours of physically strenuous exercise, including running, jumping, bending, climbing, digging, and perhaps some swimming. Dancing was also part of the routine, but probably not every day.

Stone Age man was fitter than the average westerner is today. Even a very athletic present-day person would have trouble keeping up with the prehistoric hunting group during hour-long hunts; probably only an Olympic-level endurance athlete would be able to do so. But in a clan of prehistoric hunter-gatherers, every individual between puberty and old age (yes, including females) would be able to pursue prey on foot, walking, jogging, and running for several hours at a time. The next day would be spent at rest. We know all this by observing present day hunter-gatherer societies.

Do you honestly think that with this level of regular exercise and activity, there was even the remotest chance of obesity, high cholesterol, high blood sugar, or mood imbalances? Of course not.

Most interestingly, our emotions would also be much more positive. This is because aerobic exercise (when your heart rate is raised to almost its maximum) causes the release of endorphins, i.e., happiness hormones. Every runner knows this. It is almost impossible to experience depressing emotions while you are under the influence of endorphins. Once they wear off, usually within forty-eight hours, all you need to do is run some more. Easy!

I believe that many emotional problems, even of a long-standing chronic nature, would be reduced in severity if not resolved completely if sufficient regular exercise were engaged in.

But how much is sufficient?

> I believe that about three hours vigorous aerobic exercise per week, divided into three to six sessions, is sufficient to keep your heart, blood sugar balance, metabolic rate, and emotions in a healthy state.

In an ideal world, you would also need to get some exposure to anaerobic activities (muscle training where your heart rate is not raised too much) such as weight lifting, gardening, or housework. Of course, if you have a job that is physically strenuous (builders, window cleaners, mechanics, etc.) your anaerobic activity is probably covered.

You would need to engage in this type of activity about two or three times per week or on a lower, on-going level in your normal every-day activities. The reason is that it builds strong muscles, and strong muscles burn more calories. Firmer muscle tone will also make you more shapely and attractive.

While anaerobic exercise would be part of an ideal exercise plan, I believe that it is probably unrealistic for most of us to incorporate this into our busy lifestyle in a formal way. As I said before, many people have jobs that involve some of it anyway, and even if we don't, we still carry the shopping, lift our children, clean the house, etc.

Finally I would like to recommend a stretching routine. Stretching releases muscle tensions and prepares your muscles for the next exercise session. It reduces the incidence of sports injuries, and it gives you a taller and more toned figure. A few minutes of stretching before and after your exercise routine (or any other time in between) is sufficient for this purpose. Three times per week is a minimum. I recommend a ten-minute routine that covers all muscle groups.

If you find all this a bit overwhelming, please be assured that exercise can be fitted into your day almost without a problem.

In a nutshell, you only need

3 hours per week aerobic (running, cycling, swimming)

30 minutes per week stretching (divided into three sessions)

Your aerobic exercise can be divided into thirty-minute sessions and done before or after work.

Your stretching can be done before bed or before or after aerobic exercise.

Building Block 4:
Light and Dark

The sun is our friend. Its rays make life on this planet possible. We just need to learn how to expose ourselves to the sun *safely*.

There are two reasons why we need regular exposure to daylight.

- For vitamin D production

- To maintain healthy sleep-wake cycles

Vitamin D

Why We Need Vitamin D

Vitamin D is needed in three ways:

- For the absorption and proper usage of calcium in the body. This affects bones, teeth, muscles, and the nervous system.

- For the proper functioning of immune cells.

- To inhibit improper cell proliferation, i.e., to prevent cancer.

Vitamin D is therefore essential for healthy bones and teeth. It also helps to keep muscles and nerves functioning properly. It protects against cancer.

A deficiency becomes apparent most easily in our immune system. Frequent colds, influenza, and respiratory infections may be due to a deficiency in vitamin D. These are most common during the darker months, when we spend less time outdoors. Maybe it's not a coincidence.

Natural Daylight and Vitamin D

It is a fact that we need to expose our skin to natural daylight in order to produce vitamin D. We can get some vitamin D from foods (fatty fish, egg yolks, and fortified foods), but it is unlikely that we eat these in sufficient amounts to cover our daily needs.

Vitamin D via Sunlight

We only need to expose our hands and face for a short amount of time in order to cover one day's needs of this vitamin. The exposure time depends on location and season. The further north you live, the weaker the sun's rays are, and so a longer exposure time is necessary. During the darker seasons, the sun's rays are also weaker and you need a longer exposure time.

Vitamin D production still takes place when your exposed skin is in the shade and not exposed to direct sunlight.

Vitamin D is *not* produced when light shines through modern window glazing as this type of glazing has inbuilt UV protection.

Sunscreens block vitamin D production.

Here are some rough guidelines for how much exposure time you need. In the UK during the winter time, those with dark skin need sixty minutes on their hands and face, while those with fair skin need thirty minutes. During the summer, those with dark need skin twenty minutes, and those with fair skin need ten minutes.

The recommended intake of vitamin D is not clearly established, but in the UK the guidelines are that the elderly and children up to the age of three should receive ten mcg per day, while all others should receive five mcg per day.

Recently it has been suggested that most of us are deficient in vitamin D, and that the so-called recommended daily allowance does not supply nearly enough.

Vitamin D can be stored in our liver. The liver is thought to have a storage capacity to supply us for about ten weeks. In other words, if you fill up your stores, you can last for ten weeks without any intake of vitamin D from daylight or food.

The bad news is that if you cover your skin with sunscreens, you either reduce or completely block the production of vitamin D. People who use sun blocking cosmetics are in danger of becoming severely deficient in this vitamin.

Therefore, to reduce the risk of skin cancer but still get the benefits of daylight, it is probably best to expose your skin to sunlight safely for a short time every day!

How long an exposure is safe depends on your skin type. Dark skin absorbs less sunlight and so can be safely exposed longer than fair skin. During the summer months ten minutes are probably sufficient for any type of skin. This amount of exposure does not increase your skin cancer risk. (On the contrary, there is mounting evidence that vitamin D is needed to protect against several types of cancer and could in the future even be used in an integrated cancer treatment protocol.)

After ten minutes you must cover up. You may use sun block, but better still is covering up with light clothing and staying in the shade.

A Word of Warning

Paradoxically, sun creams and sun blocks have been associated with an increased risk of skin cancer. Some chemicals found in these products are carcinogenic. They are cancer-causing not only on the skin, but also in other areas of the body. The same chemicals are also gender-bending. This means that they have a feminizing effect.

Please be aware that skin cancer has increased, not decreased, since the use of sunscreens. This is a fact.

Apparently, even the thinning ozone layer has nothing to do with increasing cancer rates. In Norway, a country with weak sunshine compared to most other countries, skin cancer rates have increased manifold, while Norway's ozone layer has remained unchanged during that same period.

Please open your eyes to the possibility that sunscreen use is one of the factors contributing to cancer.

Please also consider the possibility that skin cancer is caused by a whole host of factors, of which sun exposure is only one. Other factors may be excessive use of sunscreen, inheritance, a diet low in anti-oxidants, exposure to carcinogenic toxins, etc.

The only way to protect yourself against the part the sun plays in the causation of skin cancer is to keep out of the sun. People with many moles or fair skin and/or blue eyes should definitely avoid excessive sun exposure.

If you use anti-aging cosmetics with UV factors to reduce the appearance of wrinkles, I recommend that you think again. Reducing your natural vitamin D production will speed up aging far more than those few minutes of daylight exposure most of us get. Yes, lying in the sun for hours on end will produce leathery or crepe-type skin, but walking your dog for thirty minutes will hardly produce this effect. On the contrary, thirty minutes outdoors will be enough time for most people to produce sufficient vitamin D for one day. Even if you wear a hat and keep your face in the shade, the daylight reaching your facial skin will induce vitamin D production even whilst your skin is protected from direct sun rays. You need this vitamin D intake to keep your bones healthy and to reduce the risk of osteoporosis, a far more debilitating age-related problem than a few wrinkles around your eyes.

Safe in the Sun Whilst Inducing Vitamin D Production

Spending time outdoors in order to induce vitamin D production does not mean you will be sunbathing. Your skin will produce vitamin D even when you are in a shaded area and even on cloudy days. All that is necessary is that you are outdoors with natural daylight being able to reach your skin. A hat can protect you from direct sun rays but will still expose your facial skin to natural daylight. Sitting in the shade of a tree will allow natural daylight to reach your skin but will protect you from direct exposure.

If you must spend several hours in direct sunlight, perhaps on your children's sports day or whilst gardening, wear light, long-sleeved tops, full-length trousers, and a broad-brimmed hat. This way you will avoid the sun's harmful rays as well as the carcinogenic gender-bending chemicals in sunscreens.

I also recommend that you eat a diet rich in phyto-chemicals such as beta carotenes and anthocyanidins (found in yellow, orange, red, and blue fruits and vegetables) and rich in zinc (best supply found in meat). These nutrients help your skin to protect itself by tanning more easily and this way blocking the harmful rays of the sun.

It has been suggested that skin that is used to regular exposure to the sun is at less risk of skin cancer. It has even been suggested that young children's skin should be gradually introduced to regular exposure, first in the shade only, then gradually for very short periods, i.e., less than ten minutes, in direct sunlight. This way, the skin will learn how to tan and protect itself.

Sleep-Wake Cycles

The effect of natural daylight on our sleep-wake cycle is profound.

Lack of exposure to natural daylight will cause disruption to our inbuilt twenty-four hour body clock. This can have far-reaching consequences, such as increased risk of cancer and heart disease.

The earliest sign that our body-clock has become disrupted may be insomnia. Other symptoms may be blood sugar imbalances and depression, as well as bi-polar disorders.

Natural daylight needs to enter our eyes so that our body clock can re-set to a twenty-four hour rhythm on a daily basis. The light source needs to be above our heads for this to happen. Poor exposure to morning light will delay evening sleepiness. The effect is cumulative, meaning that the more days you spend in dim morning environments, the later you will feel sleepy in the evenings. For adults and teenagers, power naps in the afternoon do not negatively affect sleep-wake cycles but increase overall well-being.

In practical terms this means that you should do the following.

- Invest in some ceiling light bulbs that simulate natural daylight for winter days to keep your exposure to natural daylight even.

- Go outdoors every day, especially in the winter.

- Do not wear sunglasses (or at least reserve them just for driving and skiing), as these will dramatically reduce the amount of natural daylight hitting your retina. UVA/B damage to your eyesight is unlikely in the UK, especially if you observe the sun exposure rules stated above.

- Try to get your children and teens to go outdoors before lunchtime. Find them an outdoor sport or some other outdoor activity they enjoy, and encourage them to stick to it, especially in the darker months. (With teens this may remain wishful thinking!)

The Importance of Darkness

Interestingly, uninterrupted darkness is equally as important as exposure to daylight.

Sleep should take place in a completely darkened room. Switch of standby lights on TVs and stereos, and install black-out blinds. Even a brief exposure to light (although necessary for bathroom visits) during night/sleep time may cause small changes in our rhythm that may become apparent over long periods of time. Far more worrying are night lights and other regular sources of light in the bedroom.

The reason is that exposure to light during night/sleep hours can produce changes in our hormonal patterns, leading to increased appetite, sugar cravings, and weight gain. Even depression and an increased cancer risk have been associated with regular exposure to light during sleep hours.

Help your children learn to sleep in the dark without night lights. I realise that many children have a fear of the dark, and this is completely normal. But try to help them get over it. Sometimes flower essences can resolve this issue. Or, if all fails, you may want to have a light on for a little while and then switch it off as soon as they are fast asleep. If bathroom visits require a night light, please read on.

A Word about Nightly Bathroom Visits

If a young child (before puberty) needs to go to the bathroom every night, I suggest that you see a homeopath to try to correct this. In an ideal world nobody should have to use the bathroom at night, as we have hormones working to prevent this. But many of us still need to go, and if this is your only health issue, you should count yourself lucky.

However, children before puberty should not need to urinate at night on a regular basis. Eliminating bathroom visits will do away with the need for night lights and will reduce incidents of night-time waking too.

Building Block 5:
Water and Salt

Our body is about 80 per cent water. Water is the medium in which all our chemical reactions take place.

We therefore need to make sure we take in enough of the best quality we can find.

Unfortunately, our drinking and bathing water is one of the major sources of toxic pollution for our bodies.

Tap Water

Tap water contains a cocktail of minerals, heavy metals, oestrogen, pseudo-oestrogens, chlorine, and other carcinogenic chemicals. Each one of these comes with its own set of dangers.

- Oestrogens and pseudo-oestrogens (chemicals which mimic oestrogen in our body) cause us to have a dangerous surplus of this hormone, which can cause feminisation in males and cancer and other hormone-related problems in both sexes.

- Heavy metals damage our liver and nervous system.

- Chlorine upsets our digestive system and forms carcinogenic substances. It can also aggravate skin complaints and induce respiratory ailments such as asthma.

- Other chemicals such as BPA (found in plastic) are carcinogenic.

- Minerals such as calcium and magnesium serve to keep tap water alkaline (which is beneficial), but for the most part they cannot be absorbed or utilized by our body, as they are not attached to organic compounds.

To summarize, tap water is not a good source of water for our body.

Bottled Water

The quality of bottled mineral water depends on several factors. One is the mineral content of the source water, but more important is the container material and the length and temperature of storage. The problem is that most bottled water comes in plastic bottles. At any temperature, chemicals in the plastic leach into the water, but especially at the higher temperatures commonly found in hotter climates. Obviously, the longer the storage time, the more chemicals will leach into the water. The chemicals contained in plastic are carcinogenic. They also mimic oestrogen and so contribute to our general levels of oestrogen. This causes feminisation of males and oestrogen excess in females (leading to cancer and other hormonal problems).

Bottled mineral water is therefore not ideal, but it is better than tap water. It is certainly an alternative water supply that I recommend during periods away from home.

Filtered Water

The quality of filtered water obviously depends on the type of filter.

A simple **"Brita" jug-type filter** will filter out some chlorine and some of the other harmful substances. It is better than tap water, but certainly far from ideal.

Under-sink water filters which use large cartridges are far better. Depending on the specifications, they can filter out most of the chlorine, most of the heavy metals, and some of the other chemicals, leaving some of the calcium and other beneficial minerals in the water.

Provided you chose a good quality filter, these under-the-sink type solutions are a good alternative.

In my opinion, **reverse osmosis** filters are the best solution. These under-the-sink units can be quite large, but this is a compromise worth making when it comes to your health.

A reverse osmosis unit works by forcing tap water through a porous membrane, which lets through (almost) nothing but water molecules. About ninety-nine per cent of all non-water molecules are left behind in the filter.

A word of caution:

> Some reverse osmosis units are too efficient! They take out all the minerals and so produce pure water. This type of water, before it reaches your mouth, attracts chemicals from the environment that make the water acidic! Drinking water should never be acidic, as this can cause serious problems in the long run. (See the section on nutrition and keeping your body alkaline in Building Block 1.) I recommend a reverse osmosis unit by www.freshwaterfilter.com. This unit produces slightly alkaline water.

There are some **alkalising/ionising water treatment units** on the market. They claim to filter the water, but they are far too small to be able to do this. Additionally, I would avoid alkalising my water beyond 7.5ph. I believe this may be just as bad as drinking water that is too acidic, i.e., below 6.8ph.

Daily Intake

Your daily intake of water should be between one and two litres (four to eight beakers) for adults. Exercise, hot weather, high salt intake, and breastfeeding may increase your needs, but probably not beyond three litres. Most people adjust their intake naturally, as they are guided by their natural thirst.

However, it is worth keeping an eye on your intake for a while to see whether your natural thirst is guiding you correctly.

People at risk from subtle dehydration (before it becomes a life-threatening condition) are the elderly and children. Many elderly people have lost their natural thirst guidance and many children are "too busy" in their games to notice, but most people can rely on their thirst to guide them.

Although there is natural variation in what people need, if your thirst or the lack of it becomes extreme, I strongly recommend that you investigate.

Extreme thirst may indicate diabetes, and extreme lack of thirst may indicate other problems. If your doctor finds nothing wrong, you can rest assured that the problem is minor. In this case I would recommend that you try alternative methods and therapies to bring your body and thirst indicator back to a normal range.

Other Fluids

Our body does not need any other drinks than water. It does, however, need fluids contained in juicy fruit and vegetables. It is this juicy flesh of vegetables and fruit that carries the valuable vitamins, minerals, and phytochemicals we so desperately need. In fact, a diet high in conservatively cooked vegetables and fresh fruit will induce less thirst than a diet low in these foods with high water content. In the same way, a diet high in salt will induce more thirst than a diet low in salt.

A Word of Caution

Tea (even green tea), coffee, and alcoholic beverages are dehydrating! If you drink any of these, you may need even more water. In addition, these drinks reduce the amount of minerals available to your body. Alcohol reduces magnesium, zinc and vitamin B levels in a major way.

Fizzy drinks are definitely not part of a healthy lifestyle and should only *occasionally* be indulged in by adults, and never by children or teens. In particular, beware of diet versions! Artificial sweeteners are carcinogenic; they increase the risk of brain tumours. So have the honest sugar version, if you must.

Children should never be allowed to drink ordinary tea, coffee, alcohol, or fizzy drinks. Once your child is hooked on any of these, you will have trouble getting them off. So it is best to never even start.

Cola drinks contain far too much sugar, carcinogenic chemicals, addictive substances, blood sugar disrupters, stimulants, colourings, flavourings, etc. Fanta and other lemonades are not much better.

If you want to treat your child with food and drink, let them have a hot chocolate or some other honest sweet item, like a good quality ice cream, continental chocolate, or home-baked cake. At least you know what is in those, and you pretty much contain the damage to plain sugar and fat.

Bathing Water

When we sit in the bath, we absorb a considerable amount of water through our skin. It can be as much as one pint every fifteen minutes. With the water, we absorb some of the toxic chemicals too. There is no need to become obsessed about this, but if you suffer from a chronic skin condition (especially children who tend to have baths and not showers) or if you want to go the extra mile with your health bank account, I recommend that you install a whole-house water filter. This filter removes about ninety-eight per cent of all toxic chemicals but leaves healthy minerals in the water. It is available from www.freshwaterfilter.com

Salt

Salt is an essential nutrient. Its most prominent role in the body is to control the movement of water between body compartments and between our body and the outside. It is also involved in conducting nerve impulses. It is needed in every cell of our body. In fact, the importance of salt is so great and its presence so universal that Patrick Holford (a prominent nutritionist) in one of his lectures once referred to humans as "hairy bags of salty soup". Not too attractive, but certainly true.

An excess of salt is problematic, as this is thought to cause high blood pressure.

A salt deficiency is unlikely, as our body is made to retain salt. Humans have a salty tooth (as well as a sweet one), because salt is rare in natural foods yet so important in our body. Therefore our taste buds crave it, and our kidneys work hard to retain every miniscule bit of it.

For this exact reason, a diet high in salt is not desirable, because our body will retain most of it due to its evolutionary programming that was established a long time ago when salt was rare.

Once we retain too much salt, water follows. This is how some types of oedema come about. (Other types of oedema are due to hormonal imbalances.)

The biggest problem with salt, however, is not the quantity but the quality. Refined salt, which is the very fine-grained variety most of use every day, has had most of its other trace minerals removed and is almost pure sodium chloride. It also has many additives not listed on the label, as these are traces of chemicals left over from the refining process. In addition, anti-caking agents supply you with a dose of ammonium and/or aluminium compounds, all of which are toxic in our system. This type of salt is far more likely to cause damage and chronic disease than unrefined natural sea salt.

Unrefined sea salt is a mixture of many trace minerals, all essential in our body. There are some reports that unrefined sea salt that is free from anti-caking agents helps to alkalise your body and therefore improve conditions such as high blood pressure, allergies, and other chronic ailments. Try to find a variety that is free from anti-caking agents. www.celticseasalt.com stock this kind of salt.

Daily Requirement

Our daily requirement of salt is very low in spite of its importance. We need only a few grams, and we should definitely not have more than six grams per day. Ordinary table salt should not be used at all. Unrefined sea salt can be used with caution.

And again, a diet high in fresh vegetables and fruit and low in processed and pre-cooked foods is naturally low in salt and so much better from this perspective also.

Building Block 6:
Handling Pollution

Our planet is heavily polluted. Chemical toxins are found in the breast milk of mothers living on remote pacific islands. Even space is full of discarded satellites orbiting mother earth.

What to do?

> Do not get obsessed, but do become aware and decide what to avoid and where to concede.

> Please remember your health bank account. A body fortified with healthy food, sufficient sleep, and regular exercise will be well equipped to withstand some amount of pollution for many years.

> We need to identify the potential sources of pollution that can enter and damage our bodies. Only then can we make decisions as to which ones we can reasonably avoid or at least reduce.

Two Types of Toxins

One type—**endogenous**—are chemicals that are produced *inside* our body *by* our body. For instance, the breakdown and use of proteins produces a substance that must be eliminated swiftly, or it will damage body tissues and eventually lead to death.

Our body has mechanisms to handle all of these endogenous toxins, and so we should not need to worry about them. We only begin having problems if our detoxification mechanisms are not working properly. In its extreme, this is an emergency situation that will not escape the attention of any doctor.

However, a more subtle process is more common. It is one of the tenets of alternative medicine that modern day living leads to gradually worsening damage to our detoxification mechanisms. This causes a backlog of toxins inside us, which subsequently leads to disease. In the eyes of alternative medicine, chronic disease is almost always preceded by this process. The detoxification pathways can become damaged by poor diet and lifestyle habits, as well as by environmental toxins.

Of course, we may be born with a slight disadvantage in this area if we have a so-called weakened constitution. In the eyes of many alternative medicine practitioners, most people walking the planet today are born with a weakened constitution and are therefore at a disadvantage right from the start. This would partially explain why many chronic complaints start soon after birth.

The second type of toxin is called **exogenous**. These are environmental toxins, and they include anything added to our body from the outside. They may reach us via food, drink, air, water, medicines, cosmetics, soaps, hair dyes, sunscreens, recreational drugs, radiation, and so on.

These toxins are substances that our body is not designed to handle above a certain threshold (or in some cases not at all). The consequence of ingestion or inhalation of these toxins, however, is rarely instant death, but usually acute poisoning symptoms or subtle chronic ailments, which in the long run may lead to death.

Exogenous toxins are usually tackled by the same mechanisms as endogenous, and some are eliminated this way.

Even toxins that have been eliminated may leave behind some damage that our body may not be able to repair. Some are isolated in our fatty tissues, where they cannot cause any further damage. Some are caught within cells and have no way out and so continue damaging cellular components. Some alter the structure of our DNA, and some alter how our DNA is used or expressed. (This is how cancer is thought to start.)

Cocaine for instance (see below) changes the expression of our DNA to "addictive type", causing the person to become easily addicted *per se*—i.e., addicted to many other substances or even behaviours, not just cocaine. It is now thought that this type of damage or alteration may be inherited on to the next generation. Therefore, exogenous toxins may be far more dangerous than we allow ourselves to admit.

However, the human body seems to be amazingly resilient. Considering the amount of abuse I have described, we are on the whole still doing fine.

I believe that maintaining your good health is possible with a little bit of discipline and the judicious application of my recommendations. I also believe that even if you do suffer from a chronic ailment, an improvement or even a complete reversal may be possible. But for this you need to be committed and determined.

Let us now consider the different sources of exogenous toxins.

Food and Drink

Organic Food

Pesticides and artificial hormones are harmful, even if vested interests tell you otherwise. Organic food may not be entirely toxin free, but it will definitely be lower in toxins than non-organic food. If you can afford it, make sure you have as much of your food in the organic version as possible.

I would emphasise that of all foods, meat and dairy are most polluted as animals store toxins in their fatty tissues and pass these on to us.

As I explained in the nutrition section above, I do not recommend dairy as a food. If you avoid dairy, you will reduce your exposure to artificial hormones considerably. Do not underestimate this! Dairy has been associated with an increased risk of cancer.

So to summarize, eat organic as much as possible.

The highest standard of "organic" is "Soil Association" approved food and drink.

Preservatives, Flavourings, Colourings

These are mostly toxic. Some are natural or nature-derived, but they can still be toxic. It is unrealistic to completely avoid these, but try to reduce exposure by eating mostly home-made meals, with very few commercial sauces, dressings, or ready-to-cook foods.

Frozen and Tinned Foods

Frozen vegetables can be high in nutrient contents, but they still taste different to fresh varieties. It is for this reason that I am suspicious and do not recommend frozen vegetables. Frozen fish and meat are probably fine, but please use just plain varieties and no ready-made meals.

Tinned foods supply you with chemicals that leach from the tin into the food. These are carcinogenic, and so tinned food should be avoided.

Fizzy Drinks

Avoid fizzy drinks at all costs. Please refer to the water and nutrition sections above.

Also avoid the diet versions. Artificial sweeteners are carcinogenic.

Cooking Materials and Food Containers

Tefal and other coatings are carcinogenic if even the least bit scratched. Never use a coated pan with scratches! Aluminium pans are also toxic, as the aluminium leaches into food and attacks your nervous system. The least toxic option is stainless steel.

Plastic wraps and plastic food containers are carcinogenic and gender-bending. BPA contained in plastic leaches into the food, in particular into fatty foods. Please avoid these altogether.

Your children's lunchboxes and water bottles should be made from stainless steel or BPA-free plastic.

Please be aware that this is a big problem when it comes to infants and toddlers who eat and drink everything out of plastic! Investigate BPA-free bottles and containers on the internet.

Water

This is a major source of pollution for us. Please invest in a good quality filter. See the sections on water and salt above.

Air

Our air is heavily polluted. City air is worse than country air.

If you can, move to a less polluted area. Other than this, you obviously cannot avoid this source of pollution.

But you can take certain measures to reduce its impact on your body. One measure would be to eat a diet high in brightly coloured vegetables and fruit. These foods contain phytochemicals which act as "anti-oxidants", protecting your cells from damage. If your exposure to toxic air pollution is extremely high, I recommend a high quality anti-oxidant supplement on top of a diet high in vegetables and fruit as described above. This gives you extra insurance.

You can also invest in a good quality air filter and ioniser to set up in your bedroom and switch on at night. This will give you some valuable protection during your sleep.

Furniture and Fabric Out-Gassing

Many types of fabric, furniture, and decorating materials are treated with or contain toxic gasses that are continuously released into the air in your home.

There are some non-toxic varieties around, and this is worth investigating. Non-toxic paints and floor treatments are available, but fabrics and mattresses are hard to find as they are required to be treated with fire-resistant chemicals.

With regards to this type of pollution, there is a danger that you will probably just get obsessed and worried about things you cannot do much about. I recommend that you let this area go and just make sure you air out your home every day several times top to bottom and inside out.

Cleaning Materials, Detergents, Cosmetics, Perfumes

Cleaning materials are quite toxic, and to a great degree they can be avoided. There is no need to use bleach or other chlorine-based or ammonia-based cleaning materials on a regular basis. They are damaging to your airways. If your loo looks too bad after three months or so, just go ahead and use bleach once and be done with it. In between, you can use a green-label toilet cleaner, which admittedly does not do a perfect job but is acceptable for a while.

For other cleaning, there are some very good cleaning cloths available that produce a wonderful sheen without any chemical products! We must get away from our obsession with germs around the house. There is no need to disinfect every corner; in fact a bit of dirt is good for our immune system.

Your clothes and linen do not need *fabric softeners*. Detergent is sufficient. The chemicals and perfumes in these materials are toxic, and you will breathe them in continuously all day long. If you want to go the extra mile, use an environmentally friendly detergent, or even better, an "eco ball", which allows you to wash without detergent.

<u>*Cosmetics, soaps, and shampoos*</u> are a major source of toxic pollution to your body. I cannot emphasise this enough. Lathering agents in soap and shampoos are carcinogenic. The so-called natural ones derived from coconut are better, and so it is worth making the switch to organic soaps and shampoos. Also, you can use less! You do not need to shampoo your whole body every day. Just wash the smelliest bits.

Do not use antiperspirants, as they cause breast cancer, even in men! If you have to, use deodorants of the organic variety. They work, but not as efficiently. I realise that going without deodorant is unrealistic and unthinkable for most people, but at least try to get away from thinking of the natural odour of your skin as disgusting. Actually, it is this natural odour which attracts the opposite sex! So let us keep it subtle but let us keep it.

Perfumes are another source of pollution. They can damage your lungs. If you like to use scents, try to use aromatherapy oils, such as rose or jasmine. Jasmine has just been found to have natural calming effects to the same level as valium!

Cosmetics and make-up are all toxic. They actually harm your skin and cause premature aging, something you then want to correct by using more of them! If you wish to use make-up, use a less toxic variety such as Dr Hauschka or Arbonne. There are quite a few of these available now. And try to use less.

Face and body creams are entirely unnecessary and supply you with more toxins. They do not help dry or blemished skin, as these problems are caused from the inside (except in the case of contact dermatitis). If you still wish to use these products, I suggest using organic or toxin-free varieties. Plain olive oil (virgin) is a very good body moisturiser. It is not greasy, and it also has antibacterial and antifungal properties.

Hair Dyes

These are very toxic, causing bladder cancer. Permanent dyes are worse than semi-permanent. Yes, very depressing news indeed! And the worst part is that there is no way out. I suggest you use herbal semi-permanent hair colours for as long as possible. If you are feeling brave, go cold turkey and avoid toxic chemicals in hair colours altogether. White is the new blonde!

If you cannot do this, make a decision and let this area go. Visit your favourite salon and rejoice in your newly found youth. For at least two days after the salon visit, you should drink plenty of water (two litres or more) to flush the toxins out of your bladder. As always, a diet high in anti-oxidants may provide you with some protection.

Feminine Hygiene

Tampons leach toxic chemicals into your body. These chemicals attack some of your most vulnerable parts—your reproductive organs. If you want to use tampons, please invest an extra penny and use "Natracare" products. These have a reduced chemical load.

If you are able to, or want to go the extra mile, there are some very nice washable pads available. With these you avoid the problem altogether. I admit that this is not an attractive option, but I just wanted to let you have the information.

A Final Word on Beauty Products

You may not believe me at this point in time, but eating a healthy diet (as described above), exercising regularly, exposing yourself to natural daylight, and getting sufficient sleep will most likely make your body less smelly and more beautiful from the inside out than any lotion and potion can do from the outside. Your skin tone and texture will improve, and you will begin liking yourself more the natural way.

If you still have skin problems or suffer from excessive sweating after several months of employing the above measures, you may want to use various alternative therapies to tackle these problems.

Medical Drugs

Medical drugs may be necessary, but they still contain toxic chemicals that our liver must process.

Most medical treatments are based on the belief that an illness must be opposed, i.e., conquered. This is usually done with something that either poisons the invading germ or chemically alters some part of our body. Once these agents have done their part, they leave a toxic residue behind. Some of these toxins are eliminated, but some are not. Even those that are eliminated may leave some parts of your body forever changed. My recommendation is therefore to be extremely cautious when it comes to medical drugs.

Avoid all over-the-counter medication. Most of these medications are for complaints that go away by themselves in the same amount of time. We just like to feel we are doing something, and this is what these products are for. In fact, most of these medications are doing harm in your body. They suppress your symptoms and leave a toxic residue. They enable you to go on pretending that you are fine, when actually your body has been giving you a warning.

If you have a cold, you should rest more and eat a healthier diet—not take paracetamol and carry on burning the candle at both ends. If you are constipated or suffer from indigestion, you should change your diet and lifestyle—not carry on regardless. If you keep doing what you are doing, the symptoms will always come back.

At some point you will get worse, as your body has exhausted itself. Many people do not recognise this. The following example is common. Someone might say, "I used to get many colds, but not anymore. My immunity has definitely improved." When you inquire further, you find out that now they suffer from hay fever, which they never used to get. In fact, this shows that their immunity has got worse; now they are suffering from a constant cold that lasts all season! On the same note, it has recently been established that excessive usage of paracetamol in early childhood increases the risk of respiratory allergies later on in life. So be careful.

If you have a minor recurring problem, I recommend that you use alternative medicine to solve it. Alternative medicine uses energy healing or natural substances that work with your body, not against it. These substances do not leave toxic residues in your body, and they do not alter the way your body works.

If you need to take pharmaceuticals because you are in constant pain or would not be able to live without them, this is a different story. Of course these drugs still have negative effects in your body, as exemplified by their numerous side effects, but obviously you rely on them, and they cannot be taken away.

However, there are instances where a healthier diet, some specific supplements, or other alternative therapies can improve your well-being or even your symptoms. In addition, the side-effects the drugs may be reduced. So even if you have a chronic ailment that needs regular pharmaceuticals, it is worth investigating your options as to what else you might do to improve your general health and/or your condition. Please refer to the next building blocks for further information.

Recreational Drugs

Without exception, recreational drugs are absolute killers of health and well-being on the physical, mental, and emotional level. There is no compromise at all on this one.

Do not believe anyone who claims that marihuana is harmless. Paranoia sets in at a subtle level even after a few uses. Stopping the habit *does not reverse the changes* that have taken place.

Cocaine alters your gene expression to "addicted personality". This gene expression cannot be reversed by conventional methods and is now thought to be inherited on to the next generation. So by indulging yourself, you are screwing up your innocent children as well. As far as I know, only the most stringent application of naturopathic healing therapies (a combination of homeopathy, chiropractic, nutrition, and emotional healing) may be able to reverse this gene expression back to non-addictive personality.

I do not need to discuss every single drug. They all alter your brain chemistry in such a way that you do not feel okay unless you keep up the habit. They also damage your liver and ruin your life.

If you are using recreational drugs, you must stop.

Tobacco Smoking

The same applies to smoking.

However, I do believe that some people with very strong constitutions and an exemplary lifestyle in other respects may tolerate a moderate amount of smoking. But since most smokers also indulge in other ways, this scenario is highly unlikely, and so stopping smoking is the best option.

This may not be easy but there are various techniques and therapies available that can make it possible.

Radiation

Nuclear radiation is obviously unavoidable if and when it occurs. There are some homeopathic remedies that have a reputation for protecting against and healing damage caused by nuclear radiation to some degree.

Do not live near a nuclear power station.

Electromagnetic radiation is a concern in the age of the computer. We are all wired up and irradiated all day long. Most of this is unavoidable. And surprisingly, in spite of the hype surrounding this, most of it is harmless. The radiation emitted by a wireless hub reduces by something like fifty per cent by the time you have stepped one meter away. It is not strong to start with, and at a small distance it is negligible.

Mobile phone masts emit radiation, but again this type of radiation does not pass through brick or concrete, only glass and air, and so you are mostly protected unless you are passing by on foot or standing in front of your window with a mast very nearby.

Your computer screen and hardware emit radiation, but this has been minimized.

I know people who have been sitting on banks' trading floors surrounded by literally hundreds of screens and hardware in the midst of cables and wires for years! The incidence of cancer is no higher in these people than in the general population.

However, we must be aware that electromagnetic radiation is health-eroding and can be damaging. But since there is not much we can do about it without becoming seriously eccentric, I recommend taking some common sense precautions and relaxing about the rest.

- Switch off your computer, mobile phone, and stand-by buttons at night, especially if they are anywhere near your bedroom.

- Do not use a radio alarm clock, but a battery-powered one. These emit less radiation.

- Do not live under or very near a mobile phone mast and **never** under or near an electricity pylon.

- Do not live near a nuclear power station

- Reduce the time spent talking on your mobile or cordless telephone.

- Do not sleep on an electric blanket. Use a hot water bottle instead.

- Avoid routine x-rays, scans, MRIs, CTs, etc.

Again, if your body is fortified by a healthy diet and positive lifestyle as described above, you bank account is well in credit, and you can relax about radiation (as long as you observe the common-sense measures above).

If you are still concerned, I recommend you consult a homeopath who can prescribe certain remedies that have the reputation of giving some protection against radiation.

For the more superstitious there are some gadgets that claim to balance out electromagnetic radiation in your home and/or on your body. You may want to invest in one and so give yourself peace of mind.

Microwave Cooking

Your microwave cooker is your worst enemy. Microwaved food becomes denatured, as the electrical charges of food particles become disturbed. The food loses all health-giving properties, and you might as well eat paper. Do not use it.

Microwaving baby's milk bottles or pre-cooked frozen food should be stopped immediately.

Please sit down and work out a time schedule that allows you to have ten minutes extra to warm up your child's milk. And frozen food can be taken out of the freezer the night before.

Summary

Do not panic, and do not become obsessed. This in itself will make you ill. I recommend that you become aware of the potential hazards and decide where in your own personal life you can avoid toxic exposure and where you cannot. Think of your bank account, and pay in some more credit in areas where you are able to make up for toxin exposure. You may want to sleep a bit more or eat a healthier diet. Alternative medicine may help you keep your detoxification mechanisms strong. I highly recommend integrating some form of treatment into your life to adjust your body on a regular basis. And of course this would be part of the credits you are paying into your heath bank account. Then lean back, rest assured, and turn your mind to more pleasant thoughts.

Building Block 7: Medicine

A discussion about health has to include a discussion of medical therapies and the art of healing.

Even when we look after ourselves to the best of our abilities, there will be times when we get ill or when we somehow do not feel right. Or perhaps we suffer from a chronic ailment that cannot be resolved with lifestyle measures alone.

This is when we need to use some form of medical therapy or treatment to improve our well-being.

It is my conviction that if you are a layperson—and most people are—you should definitely consult with a registered medical doctor in the first instance. You should also do this if you consider yourself not a layperson, unless the complaint is so minor that it can be assumed to be harmless. Examples of such minor complaints are colds, mild headaches, mild allergic reactions to insect bites, mild constipation, and the like. But if in doubt, or if a complaint recurs or carries on for a long time, you must consult with a medical doctor.

Medical doctors have the best training in diagnosis and also have the best facilities at hand. Of course, they are only human, and sometimes they make mistakes, but on the whole you are in safe hands, at least when it comes to finding out what your problem is.

If your problem is of the more severe category, I recommend you get several opinions. I realise that for this you may need to consult privately, but I believe that your health is worth this expense, especially when it comes to perhaps preventing an unnecessary operation or a lengthy medical drug treatment.

You may also consult a respected alternative medical practitioner to give you another perspective on your problem. This can sometimes be an eye opener, but for severe problems it is only appropriate *after* you have obtained a correct medical diagnosis.

Once you are indeed sure that the diagnosis is correct, you are free to proceed as you wish. It remains your own responsibility how you want to address your problem.

If you are the guardian of a minor, I recommend that you take this whole process very seriously indeed. And by this I mean that you should get at least three medical opinions and two alternative ones. This obviously applies to anything extremely serious, such as cancer and heart disease, but also to less serious procedures such as removing tonsils and circumcision due to recurring infections.

Once you are sure of the diagnosis you must make a decision as how to proceed.

These are your options:

- Do nothing.

- Follow the conventional medical route exclusively.

- Combine conventional medical treatment with alternative therapies.

- Follow the alternative route exclusively.

I believe that the route you chose must depend on the nature of the complaint.

Some complaints need no treatment. They go away by themselves. If they recur several times, it is time to seek advice.

Alternative practitioners are prohibited by law from treating some complaints. These include cancer, diabetes, tuberculosis, venereal infections, and several infectious diseases. However, an alternative practitioner is allowed to give you treatment *while* you suffer from these complaints, but only for your general well-being or to help with side-effects of medical treatments.

All remaining complaints can be addressed simultaneously by medical and alternative treatments. Examples are skin complaints, respiratory complaints, digestive complaints, hormonal problems, heart problems, depression, anxiety, etc.

Some complaints are not life-threatening and therefore can be treated safely with alternative medicine alone. These include ear-nose-throat infections, mild to medium severity chest infections, headaches (as long as sinister causes have been excluded), skin complaints and skin infections, digestive complaints (except acute emergency situations of intestinal blockage and appendicitis), female complaints (fibroids, endometriosis, PCOS, PMS, period problems, infertility), male complaints, ME, fibromyalgia, arthritis, insomnia, ADHD, learning disorders, and delayed development.

This list is not complete, but it covers the most common ailments that can be treated safely with alternative medicine alone. It is, however, always recommended to get a medical diagnosis first to exclude sinister and life-threatening situations that may lurking in the background.

What Exactly Are Alternative Therapies?

Any therapy that does not belong to the mainstream medical system is an alternative therapy.

The most popular and well-known are:

- acupuncture

- aromatherapy

- Ayurveda

- Chinese medicine

- chiropractic

- healing

- herbal medicine

- homeopathy

- hypnotherapy

- kinesiology

- massage therapies of various nature

- NLP

- nutritional therapy

- osteopathy

- reflexology

Psychotherapy, psychoanalysis, and counselling (of various schools) are therapies that are often used by mainstream medicine but that do not employ pharmaceutical drugs.

We shall now consider the various benefits of alternative treatments.

The Benefits of Alternative Treatments

No Harmful Side-effects

Good alternative treatments do not have any harmful side-effects. Some treatments, such as osteopathy, chiropractic, healing, massage, acupuncture, etc., are of a purely physical manipulative nature and so cannot possibly produce chemical side-effects. Other treatments, such as homeopathy, herbal medicine, Chinese medicine, Ayurveda, etc., use only natural medicines (non-pharmaceuticals) in a very controlled fashion.

Natural medicines can be very toxic too and can also have side-effects, but in alternative therapies these substances are used in a way that should exclude this possibility.

Of course, a practitioner may be poorly trained or make mistakes, (and this happens to medical doctors too), but on the whole, instances of actual harm coming out of any alternative procedure are rare. What is more common is that the therapy does not produce the desired effect.

To be safe, I recommend that before you consult any alternative practitioner, you check their qualifications with the relevant registering professional body. Each discipline has at least one if not several professional bodies. A quick internet search will guide you to these. The best-case scenario would be to get a referral from someone you trust who has been treated satisfactorily by a particular practitioner.

Improved Immunity

Alternative therapies stimulate your inbuilt immune response. The aim is to improve your immunity and to leave you stronger and more resistant when your treatment has finished.

Conventional medicine cannot do this, since it has no mechanism or medicine that promotes immunity. Since its aim is to eradicate an infectious agent or to suppress symptoms, your immunity is usually weakened after any medical treatment. This is because your immune system is prevented from practicing! Antibiotics do away with the need for an immune response. Your immune system can go to sleep while the antibiotics do all the work for you. Calpol, too, stops a fever and thereby reduces the activity of your immune system. With repeated use of conventional medicine, it is most likely that your immune system will become lazy, untrained, and ineffective.

Alternative therapies work either by supplying raw materials which your immune system needs to get stronger (e.g., nutritional therapy) or by redirecting and concentrating the immune system's formerly diffuse efforts towards a certain goal (e.g., homeopathy). Both are valid approaches, and both may have the added benefit of leaving you in the position to get through a future incident by yourself. Alternative medicine wants your immune system to learn. Its main efforts are aimed at not disturbing it and at encouraging it to practice.

Healing Reactions

During alternative treatment, the only negative effect you may experience is a so-called healing reaction. Most commonly, there are no healing reactions, but you may just feel more tired and in need of sleep and rest. A good and experienced practitioner knows how to minimise a healing reaction so that you are only aware of it but are not suffering during it.

Healing reactions are symptoms caused by your body detoxifying or rebalancing itself. During a course of chiropractic treatment for lower backache, you may experience short intervals (a few hours at a time) of mild discomfort in your hips or neck area. This may be due to the body becoming aware of tension in these places and trying to push you into a position of no tension. While your body is finding this new healthy position, you may experience some discomfort.

Another example would be getting a mild cold during a course of homeopathic treatment for a seemingly unrelated condition. The cold allows your body to eliminate toxins through your airways carried by mucus and phlegm. This is beneficial as long as it is mild and non-debilitating.

Healing reactions, if they occur, are a vital part of your alternative treatment. Your practitioner should explain this to you and should help you move through them without anxiety. A healing reaction signifies an attempt by your body to correct its problem. It is therefore a beneficial incident and should be welcomed.

In the long run, alternative treatments fail if these healing reactions are continuously suppressed with medication. This is why good communication between patient and practitioner is paramount for alternative treatments to succeed.

Time to Talk and the Placebo Effect

Alternative therapies pride themselves on encouraging communication between patient and practitioner. Many therapies have consultations that last at least thirty minutes and are often an hour or longer. (To be fair, a consultation with a hospital consultant, medical specialist, or surgeon often also lasts at least thirty minutes. I have heard people remark favourably on this, especially after being used to fast-paced five-minute consultations with their GP. Many medical specialists also have more time and space for alternative therapies than GPs, or at least they consider that "doing nothing" may be a viable option.)

The idea behind lengthy consultations is the premise that the patient has arrived at his or her illness via a journey that started well before birth and has lasted every single day till the present. The present complaint is not isolated from the rest of the person (except perhaps in some accidents and injuries) or his or her journey, but is connected to everything medical and non-medical that is occurring presently or that has occurred previously in his or her life. Therefore the practitioner needs to have a lot of time. He needs to spend his time wisely and pinpoint relevant pieces of information. He then needs time to come to a conclusion and design a treatment plan.

Obviously this process looks slightly different for different therapies. A chiropractor, for instance, will need ten to fifteen minutes to talk to the patient about his or her medical history and then about thirty minutes to assess all the nerve reflexes and pathways. He will then take ten minutes or so to "adjust" the patient mechanically. Follow-up appointments last only about ten minutes but are very frequent, sometimes three times per week.

A nutritionist will spend at least an hour in conversation with the patient, often longer, and then will form his conclusion and design a written nutritional programme.

An acupuncturist will assess the patient physically and then insert his needles at various points.

What all therapies have in common is the idea that the patient is an individual who is completely unique and different from anyone else. Also, the patient is addressed as a whole, with all levels (physical, emotional, mental) seen as connected to each other and feeding from each other.

The result for the patient is commonly a feeling that for the first time in his life he or she has been taken seriously. Finally, someone has listened to all the seemingly unconnected nonsense and found it extremely interesting and important. No judgement seems to be passed on strange behaviours or attitudes. For the practitioner, these are all just symptoms that he needs to be told about.

In the case of mechanical therapies, this understanding comes across in the way the physical contact takes place. Massage therapists, acupuncturists, chiropractors, osteopaths, and healers all have in common an unconditional interest and acceptance of the patient's unique physical body and his or her imbalances.

It is because of this special therapeutic relationship that is formed during the alternative consultation that the idea of placebo comes to mind.

Even practitioners themselves often suspect that an element of this is present, but we tend to call it "intention". When the treatment is given with "intention", it has a better chance of success.

I recommend that if you wish to consult an alternative practitioner, you should find yourself someone with whom you have the right "vibes". You are not trying to make him or her your best pal. In fact, this is not recommended. However, it is important that the therapeutic relationship is built on trust and empathy. You must feel that the practitioner has the "intention" to help you. If you do not feel this, or if you are in any doubt, I would find another one.

The Self-Healing Capacity of Your Body

As I touched upon above, our bodies have a capacity to heal themselves. We all accept this when it comes to minor cuts and grazes. But as soon as we have a cold, we forget all about this and reach for tonics and pills. This is partially because we cannot afford to be ill and partially because we have lost the trust that we can get better without any help.

The most damaging and extreme results of this mentality are seen during childhood. Many parents simply do not have the energy or the time to allow their child to heal naturally. How can you get through stressful working days after a bout of five nights tending to your sick child? Fevers, coughs, and colds are always worst at night, and to complement this, our energy and emotional strength is usually lowest at that time too. Now imagine a family with three children, where all will go through their episodes in succession. Once they are all through, the first one will start up again. And this can go on all winter.

It is therefore easiest to reach for Paracetamol and antibiotics and be done with it. Your child is knocked out for the night, and you can sleep and go to work the next day.

What a relief!

But unfortunately, it will just happen again. And again you will reach for pharmaceutical relief. And again and again.

Some children are sick once a month all through the winter. Then, once they are between seven and nine years old, they stop. You believe that their immunity has improved, but suddenly, come April, they seem to have hay fever! They never had this before. Now you reach for antihistamines, decongestants, or even steroids, which further suppress the immune system's attempts.

This is a very common development. A medical doctor will not see any connection and will just carry on prescribing for each separate complaint and incident.

An alternative practitioner will see the connection and the path that has led to the present state.

What has happened is that the child's immune system has never been allowed to practice and build up its defensive strength. While Calpol and antibiotics do all the work, the immune system can go back to sleep. And it will. When finally it has given up trying to practice on acute infectious germs, it raises its sensitivity and starts trying to practice on everyday substances (such as pollen) that other people do not find problematic. This is because it desperately wants to do something! But now it is doing something chronic and destructive, whereas before it was actually trying to be constructive.

Only alternative medicine has the means to go back and recognise where things have gone wrong. It also has the means to do something about it in a constructive way. Alternative medicine may indeed be able to improve hay fever and it may be able to bring the immune system back to its previous state.

To return to our self-healing capacities, your child, during his regular fevers and colds does not need any medication. It has been established by several studies that antibiotics do not shorten the length of an ear-, throat-, or chest infection. The reason is that most of these are viral.

Then why do we feel better so much quicker when we take the antibiotics? Probably we don't, as we never tried without! The first time you try without will not be the first time you have an infection. Your body is therefore already in a weakened state, and it will take longer to heal by itself than if you had never had antibiotics and medicines before.

For acute infections of the ear, nose, throat, and chest I recommend homeopathic remedies. These usually reduce the pain to bearable levels almost instantly, and within twelve hours or so there should be an enormous improvement. But this is only if the correct remedy has been chosen! During the night, your child should fall asleep and wake every two or three hours. You need to repeat the remedy, and your child should go back to sleep. The whole episode should pass within a few days.

The added benefit is that homeopathy does not interfere with the immune system. It actually enables the immune system to work more efficiently. It therefore gets stronger from episode to episode, making each one less severe. Additionally, episodes of infection and fever become less frequent. (When you first switch to homeopathy, you may have some backlog to clear, and healing reactions may take place.)

As a very rough guideline, from about four years onwards, a healthy child should have only about three days of fever per year plus two decent colds.

On the other hand, a child that never has a cold and never has a fever has lost the capacity to react acutely to germs. This means that at some point a chronic immune weakness will set in, such as hay fever or another allergy.

Some children are born like this, but even in those cases, alternative medicine may help to improve the immune system.

Even if it is impaired by many incidents of pharmaceutical intervention, our self-healing capacity is present till death, but in most cases it needs to be activated and guided in an intelligent way. Alternative medicine can do this for you. There are a large number of disciplines to choose from, so there is probably a therapy for everyone.

And if you think that alternative medicine is only suitable for minor infections, please read again the beginning of Building Block 7 on "Medicine". Alternative medicine has a huge range of application, either on its own or as a complement to conventional medicine. Even while you are taking pharmaceutical drugs, alternative medicine may work by stimulating and guiding the self-healing mechanisms of your body.

There are many complaints people live with unnecessarily, only because they do not know that there is an alternative! So if there is anything you would like to get rid of, please take the time to investigate. In this day and age, there is so much information to be found via the internet. Make use of it!

Even if you are not convinced, do yourself a favour and keep pharmaceuticals and other medical procedures such as cosmetic surgery, x-rays, and scans to an absolute minimum. These are really only for extreme and life-threatening situations.

Building Block 8: Emotional Well-being

Emotional well-being is probably the number one aim of us all. What good is all the talk about physical health if you are not happy?

Emotional health is very important, as our emotions influence our immune strength and our hormones. They have a profound effect on our body chemistry.

Proof for this was found by the science of epigenetics, which discovered that child abuse causes changes in the DNA expression of victims. This is how profoundly affected we are by the chemistry of our emotions.

This insight may lead us to try to influence or even control our emotions so that only positive ones emerge. We do not wish to damage our health with negative feelings!

Unfortunately, this kind of self-control is not possible. Even if you try, you will not succeed. All that will happen is that you will beat yourself up over anything negative you feel, say, and think. In other words, you will be feeling guilty, which is a negative emotion!

Negative emotions are part of life just as much as positive ones.

The key to handling our emotions lies in the following.

> Emotions pass. They are chemical reactions in your body that are very acute and then wear off within seconds, minutes, or hours. This is what happens in a healthy and adjusted individual. We often see this in young children.

However, emotions only pass if we give them an outlet. They have to be eliminated, just as any other toxic substance in our body. When we cry, we eliminate our pain. (This may be physical or emotional pain.) When we scream, we eliminate our anger. When we jump around, we eliminate our excitement. This is what children do, and this is why children return to a balanced state very quickly.

But some of these natural emotional eliminations are not socially acceptable for adults, and so we hide them, suppress them, or stuff them down with food, drink, or cigarettes, and this is exactly why we get stuck in an emotional state. We do not eliminate, but we suppress and keep within that which should be let out. This is when we do not return to normal within minutes or hours. This is when we can get stuck in some moment of hurt for a long time. And this is when emotions make us unhappy and when they make us ill by damaging our hormones and our immune system.

It would be better to find a healthy way of handling our emotions, but we cannot dance around every time we are happy, and we cannot beat up anyone who annoys us.

So what to do?

For acute emotions, I suggest you stop worrying about showing them and do what feels right to you (short of committing an offence). If you are not happy with your emotional responses, I suggest you investigate what sort of therapy might help you. There are many therapies that have an effect on emotional responses. Counselling and psychotherapy are the obvious ones, but many others, including hypnotherapy and NLP, and even homeopathy and chiropractic, can have a positive effect. These therapies may help you find a socially acceptable way of processing and eliminating intense acute emotions and thereby avoiding long-term effects from holding them in.

For chronic emotions, such as depression, anxiety, phobias, and violence, I suggest you investigate your lifestyle first, as a large proportion of mental and emotional health problems have a root in poor lifestyle choices. It is as if certain lifestyle mistakes serve to blow emotional problems out of proportion.

A comprehensive overhaul is probably necessary.

- You need to adjust your diet. Emotional health is influenced tremendously by what you eat. The main dietary culprits for emotional instability are sugar, stimulants, food additives, dairy, cereals, and alcohol.

- You need to adjust your sleep patterns. Regular and sufficient sleep is an absolute must. Lack of sleep causes mood-swings and instability.

- You need to exercise and spend some time outdoors every day. This will allow your endorphins to kick in and give you a natural boost.

- You must try to reduce your exposure to toxins and pollutants in order to improve your detoxification pathways which also eliminate your emotional chemicals.

When you have done all this for at least six months, you will realise how much of your emotional instability is simply caused by poor lifestyle choices. Some of your emotional problems may have dissolved into thin air. Some may not, and these are your real issues that you may want to treat with some kind of therapy if you feel they are definitely impairing your happiness.

On the other hand, we all have some hang-ups, some problems, or some aspects of ourselves we do not like. We do not need therapy for every little issue. Part of growing up is to accept some of our short-comings. They make us unique and give us character. So please do not get obsessed, but stay realistic.

There is no perfect human being. We all overreact sometimes, and we all get upset, angry, or excited on occasions.

I believe that constant happiness is not possible. Our emotions go up and down in perpetual motion. Find yourself a picture of the Yin/Yang symbol and reflect on it.

Building Block 9:
Spiritual Health

It is a fact that we do not know whether there is a God (or many Gods). We can only choose to believe or not.

Is it important for our general health whether we are spiritual?

It is my inclination to believe that spirituality gives life an extra dimension.

In its most positive application, spirituality seems to install calmness, acceptance, and trust. It gives us a feeling that we are being looked after, a feeling that we are not alone, a feeling that we are okay the way we are. It also seems to help us connect with the environment and nature, and, of course, it gives us empathy and charity.

Even the most entrenched atheist must admit that such emotions and attitudes will at least produce beneficial chemical reactions in our body! And, if this is all spirituality is good for, then this is enough.

The extra dimension comes in when we begin to find purpose and meaning in our lives through spirituality. We can find this without spirituality, but then our purpose may be to gain higher status, gain fame and recognition, or simply make more money. There is nothing wrong with these aims, and more often than not, they will still benefit more people than just the person who is pursuing them. Jobs will be created, inventions will come about, and progress will be made. All of this is positive for mankind.

But on a personal level, the motivation of wanting more money, more fame, and higher status comes from a place of anxiety. This anxiety may never be resolved, because there is always more to be achieved, and there are always other people who may get there first, leaving us behind!

When our purpose is fuelled by spirituality—because we believe that we are meant to do something for the common good and that we were put here to do this particular job which nobody else can do—we begin feeling calm and certain. We begin feeling that there is a place for us and that our uniqueness has earned us this place. We also understand that everyone else also has such a place and that there is no need to feel anxious or envious about our place, because there is enough for everybody.

When you feel that there is enough in every sense, you have beaten your most basic fear. This fear is your fear of survival. This fear has haunted mankind since we left paradise in the proverbial sense, i.e., since we stopped being animals and became thinking man. And this fear keeps gnawing away at our bones and tissues.

Animals never worry whether there is enough. If there is not, they go and get some more, or they die. But they do not worry about it.

Man worries day in and day out.

The problem with worrying is that it often causes us to engage in behaviours that are health-eroding. We use foods and drinks to calm us down; we take pills and potions to clear up minor ailments that we worry about too much; we have circling thoughts that prevent us from sleeping; we feel hurried and stressed; we become obsessive about cleanliness and so waste our time that we could spend exercising or resting; we have destructive relationships because we dare not be alone; and so on and so on. All these behaviours have a root in anxiety, and all of these behaviours put us on the path of gradual-onset chronic disease (as we have discussed in the chapters above).

Spirituality helps us dissolve this basic anxiety and allows us to trust and reach out.

I believe that this is the key message of any type of spiritual discipline. It does not matter what type or form of spirituality you choose. It may not even be a formal one, but one of your own making, just a sense of something spiritual.

Of course, it may be possible to find this place without spirituality, but perhaps you are just being spiritual without knowing it.

Conclusion

Human beings need certain conditions to be healthy. We have discussed these extensively. You may not agree, but at least I have got you thinking.

If you do agree, please remember the concept of your health bank account. You may not be able to implement all the above measures all the time. You may decide that some are totally against your inclinations or your taste, but at least you are now able to pick and choose. Some areas you can go the extra mile in. Those will be areas that you enjoy or that come easily to you. (Although to be healthy, you cannot cut out any area completely.)

One thing I hope has become clear: the more lifestyle measures you implement, the less you will need to use some form of medicine.

As a final word I would like to say that we should enjoy our life.

I repeat what I said at the beginning: this guide is not intended to make your life a misery. Quite the opposite. My intention is to show you how much of your health and happiness is of your own making.

I hope I have encouraged you to take some of your health into your own hands.

Biography

Maria Jevtic BSc (Hons) RSHom LCHE DNTh
Homeopath and Nutritionist

Maria is a fully qualified homeopath and a member of the Society of Homeopaths. She was awarded a BSc Honours in Homeopathy in June 2008 after completing four years of study at the Centre for Homeopathic Education. Additionally, Maria trained for two years at the Institute for Optimum Nutrition and subsequently for two years at The Plaskett College for Nutritional Medicine, where in 2001 she received her Diploma in Nutritional Therapeutics (DNTh) with distinction. Both institutes are highly respected training colleges for nutritionists.

Maria is registered with two alternative medicine professional organisations, the British Association for Applied Nutrition (BANT) and the Society of Homeopaths (SoH). Both organisations only accept practitioners with the highest professional qualifications and demand from their members a strict adherence to their ethical code of conduct.

Maria has been working as a homeopath and nutritionist for several years. She sees people in her own clinic in Wimbledon and helps babies, children, and adults improve common conditions such as eczema, acne, psoriasis, asthma, hay fever, poor immunity, female complaints, digestive complaints, sleep problems, ME, ADHD, anxiety, and depression.

Maria has previous professional experience as a classical musician. The culmination of her musical career was her seven-year membership of the viola section of the Royal Opera House, Covent Garden where she enjoyed performing many operas, ballets, and concerts.

Maria is mother to son Thomas, who has been brought up with natural remedies and without vaccinations.

Consultations are available in English or German.

Contact

Maria invites your comments and is happy to answer your queries.

maria@jevtics.net

www.familyhomeopathy.co.uk

About the Book

This book is the ultimate no-nonsense guide to taking charge of your own health. Its aim is to give you just enough high quality information to make very significant changes. The beauty of this book lies in its simplicity. The concept of health is explained with the idea of a bank account that needs to stay in credit. In order to remain healthy we must pay in daily credits and avoid too many debits. Nine building blocks of health have been identified, each explained in its own chapter. Every building block is equally important, and following Maria's simple explanations enables you to take appropriate action towards building a healthier you.